A N

is a story that is intended to reflect the feelings of those
of us who struggle with anxiety, depression, grief, anger,
doubt, shame, fear, and more, yet provide encouragement
that difficulties such as these can be helped. It expresses
how routine thoughts of negativity can sometimes cloud our
reality, making it difficult to enjoy life, to appreciate what is
truly good, to have positive relationships, or to develop to one's
full potential. It is a story that reminds us that perception is
reality. If one is willing to look, willing to accept, and willing to
try, there is a light both within and beyond available to not only
illuminate, but to change our world for the better.

Our hope is that this story and the discussion guide that follows

will become a springboard for
a conversation with ourselves
and/or with others to define
what our dark clouds are and
how we can make efforts to
find the light of our new norm.

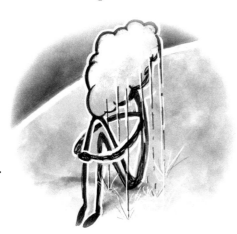

- Tom Roberts

A New Norm is the result of a partnership
between Avera and
Children's Home Society of South Dakota
in a joint effort to promote mental wellness.
Purchases of this book will benefit the mission of
helping kids and families served by
both of these organizations.

For information about how to get additional copies of this book,
go to chssd.org/books

A New Norm
Text copyright ©2018 by Tom Roberts
Illustration copyright ©2018 by Jim Brummond
Printed in the U.S.A. All rights reserved.

T&T Publishing
Sioux Falls, SD 57103
Illustration & Design by Jim Brummond
Jim Brummond - Art-Design-Photography
www.jimbrummond.com

Printed by – Sisson Printing
3500 S. Duluth Ave., SFSD 57105
Job #156672
Press Date: November 1, 2018

ISBN # 978-0-9723868-9-0

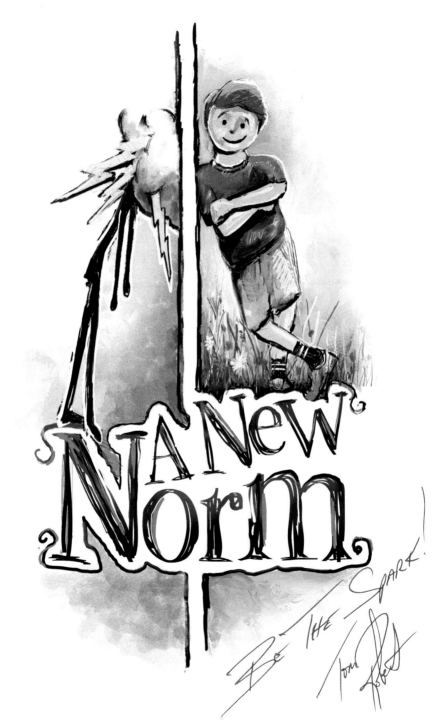

A New Norm

Be the Spark!

There once was a boy
whose name was Norm
and inside his head
Was a terrible storm

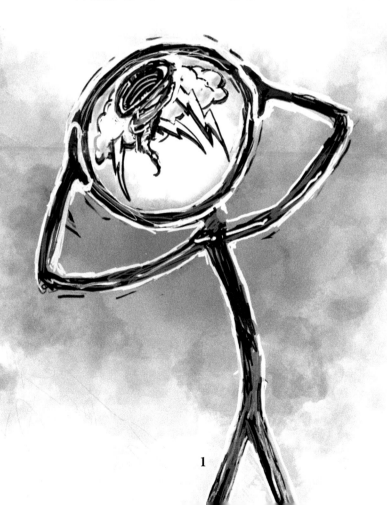

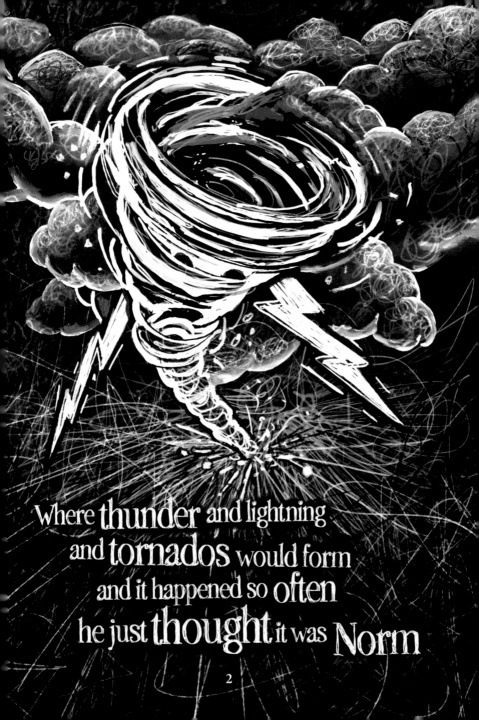

Where thunder and lightning
and tornados would form
and it happened so often
he just thought it was Norm

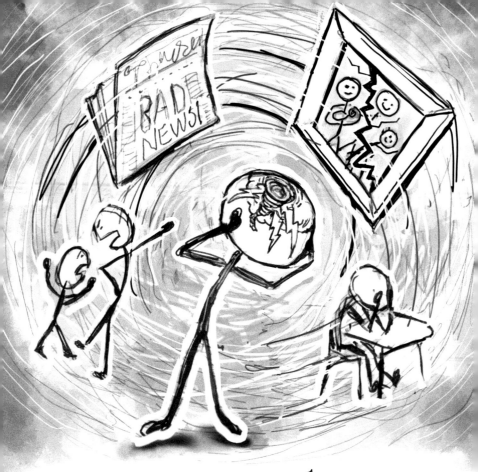

These **storms** would **happen**
whenever **there** was bad—
things that were **scary**
or **hurtful** or **sad**

But he thought it was normal when these things occur as if that was the way things always were

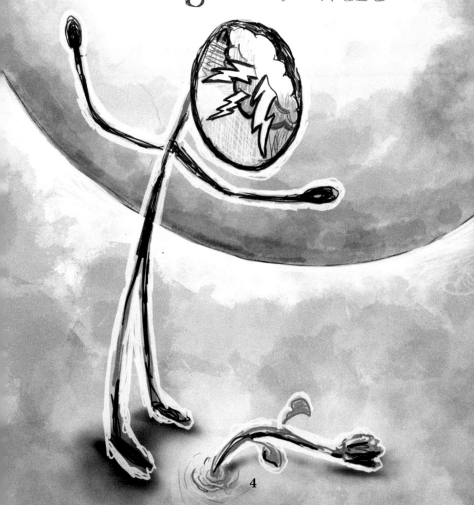

In his eyes the world was unhappy and cold just a miserable place where bad things unfold

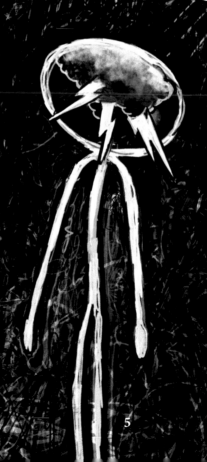

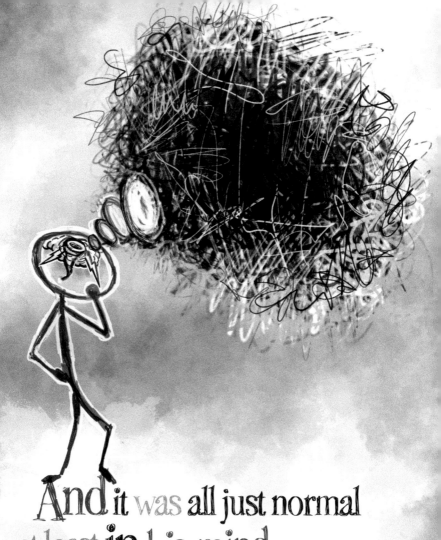

And it was all just normal
at least in his mind
that everything seemed
so dark and unkind

6

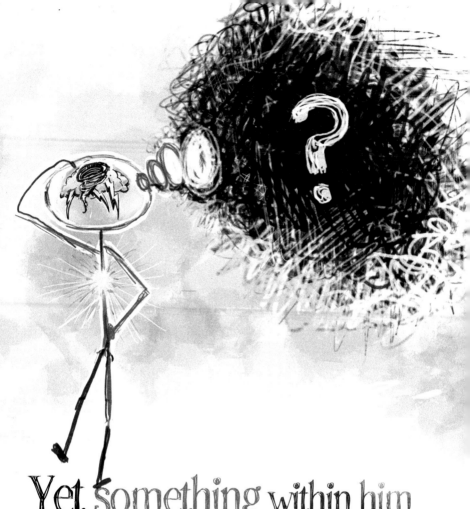

Yet something within him
something at his core
made him wonder if maybe
there was anything more

A spark of hope
that maybe there was good
where life would happen
like a good life could

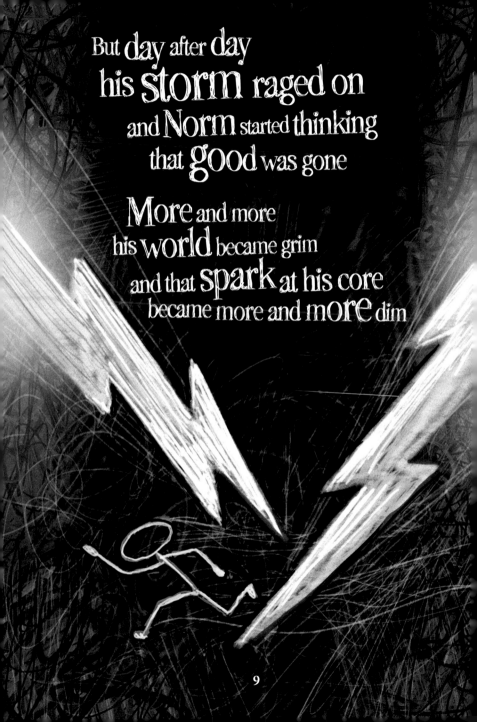

But day after day
his storm raged on
and Norm started thinking
that good was gone

More and more
his world became grim
and that spark at his core
became more and more dim

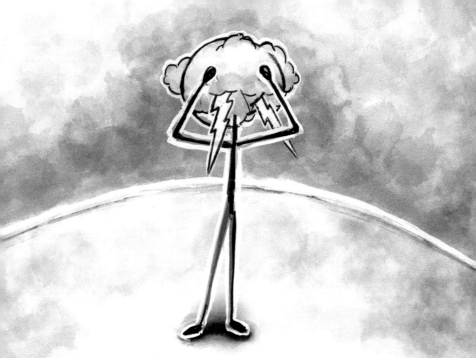

The storm inside him
began to come out
and a visible change
in Norm came about

It seems his feelings
of gloom and dread
was now creating
a cloud on his head

10

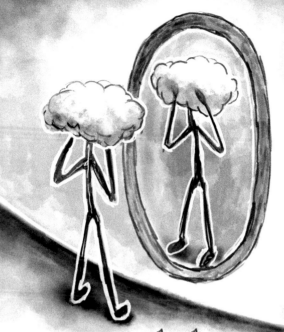

It surrounded his face
his ears and his hair
and he wondered, "Is it normal
to have a cloud there?"

It made it very hard
to see and to hear
or recognize himself
when he looked in the mirror

He tried to **shake** it off
but it would **not** shake
it just grew **bigger**
with **every effort** he'd make

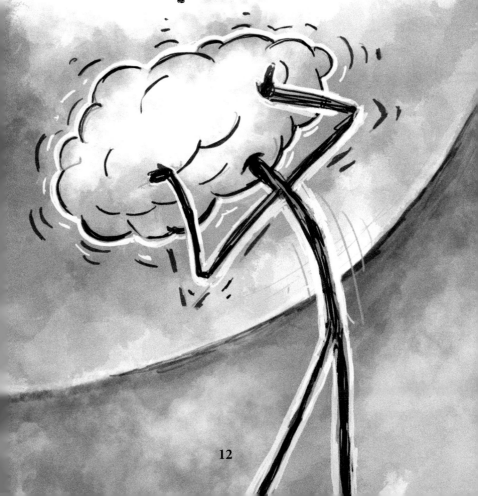

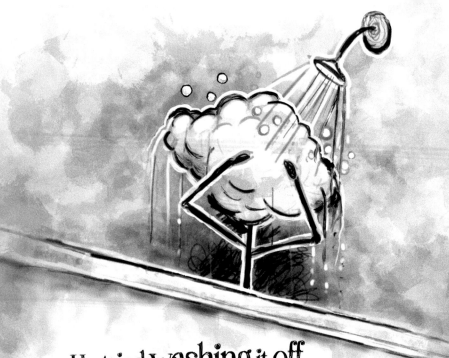

He tried washing it off
by taking a shower

and scrubbed real hard
for almost an hour

But it did not work
the cloud was still there
surrounding his face
his ears and his hair

He tried eating more pizza
and drinking more pop
But as you can imagine
that too was a flop

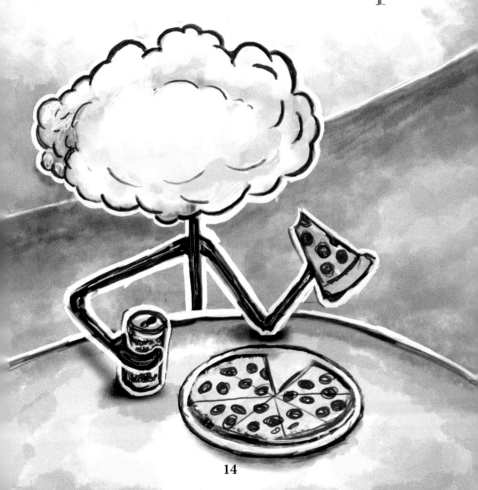

He tried yelling and shouting
and screaming real loud
but it had no effect
on that nasty old cloud

Instead it just scared
the few friends that he had
and gave them the sense
it was Norm that was bad

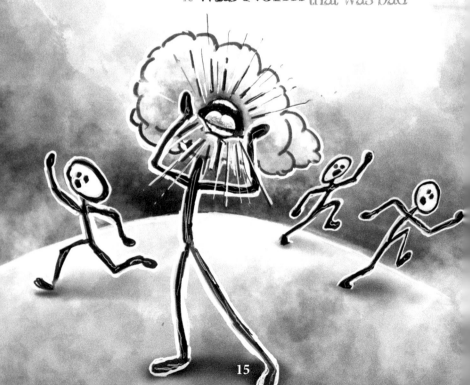

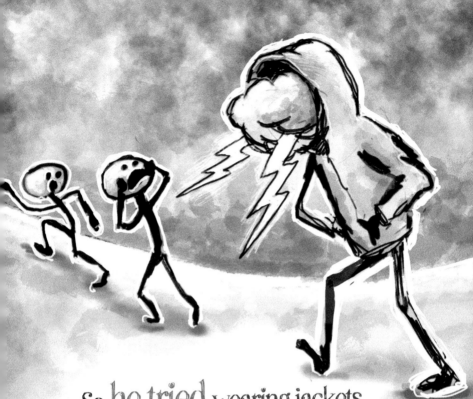

so he tried wearing jackets
(those ones with a hood)
thinking he could hide it
but it did no good

Others still saw it
and thought it was frightening
especially when it rumbled
with thunder and lightning

16

He tried running away
(a choice that was wrong)
'cause wherever Norm went
that cloud went along

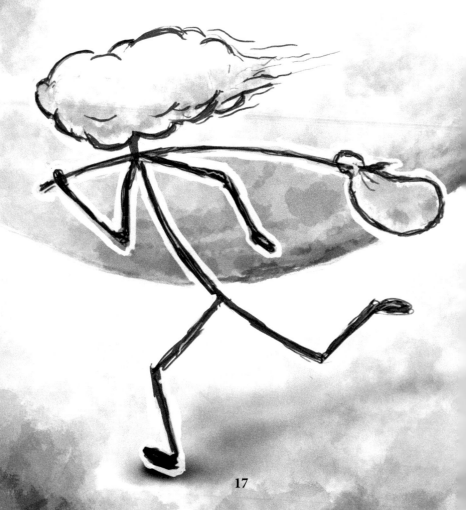

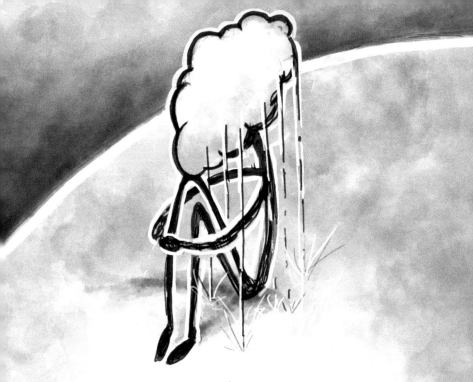

Norm was exhausted
and tired of even trying
he was tired of how that cloud
made him always feel like crying

Every day it got worse
the cloud became a wall
and Norm became numb
feeling nothing at all

He saw only darkness
he could hear only doubt
and considered giving up,
giving in or checking out

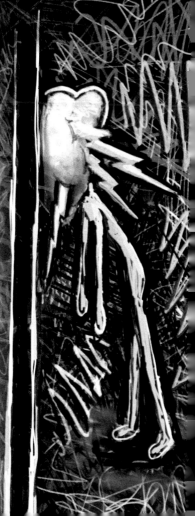

But deep down inside him
he knew it wasn't right
'cause deep down inside him
was that spark of light

And then... one day
something out of the norm
something unusual
interrupted his storm

He somehow encountered
a mysterious glow
it was a glow of goodness
and Norm wanted to know

How he could see this
through the cloud on his head
when normally he saw
only darkness instead

It was a bright light
that made its way through
the thick foggy cloud
that Norm was used to

When he closed his eyes
the light still shined
he could see it in his heart
he could see it in his mind

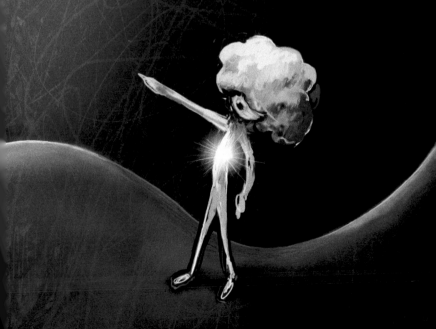

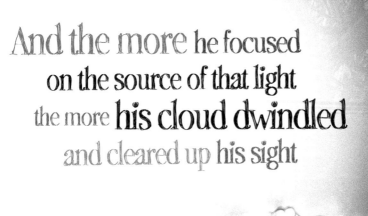

And the more he focused
on the source of that light
the more **his cloud dwindled**
and cleared up his sight

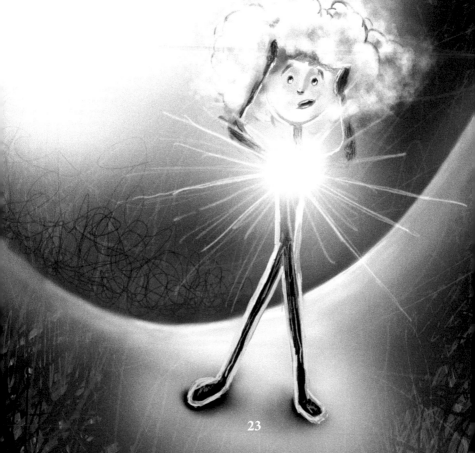

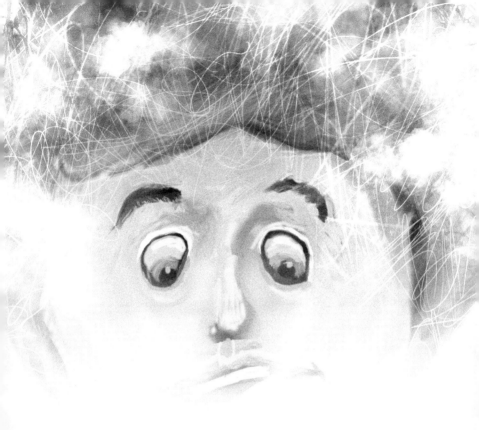

It somehow had touched
that spark deep within
which grew bigger and brighter
and he felt a change begin

The world around him
became more clear
and he saw a better normal
when he looked in the mirror

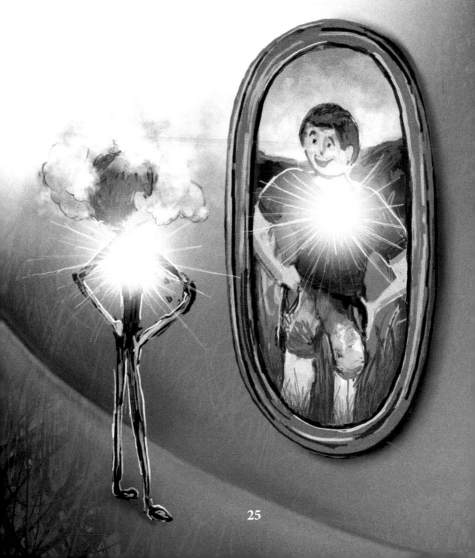

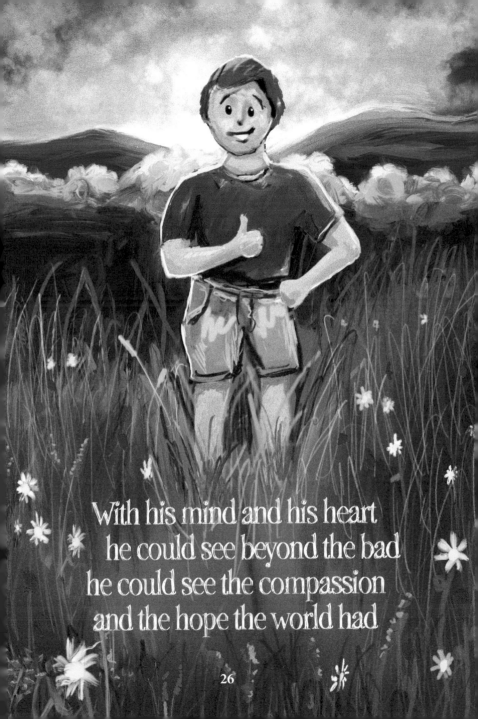

With his mind and his heart
he could see beyond the bad
he could see the compassion
and the hope the world had

26

And with this new view
he now understood
with the help of the light
he indeed could find good

Norm's life was changing
and was turning around
his cloud was fading
and more peace could be found

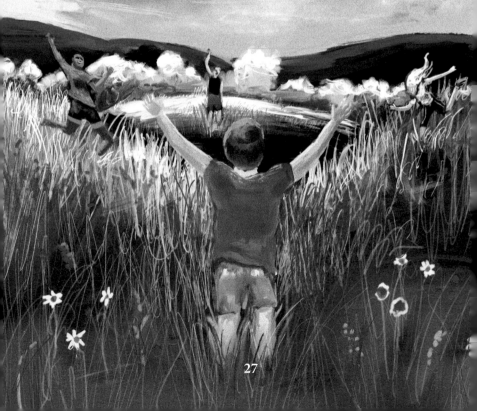

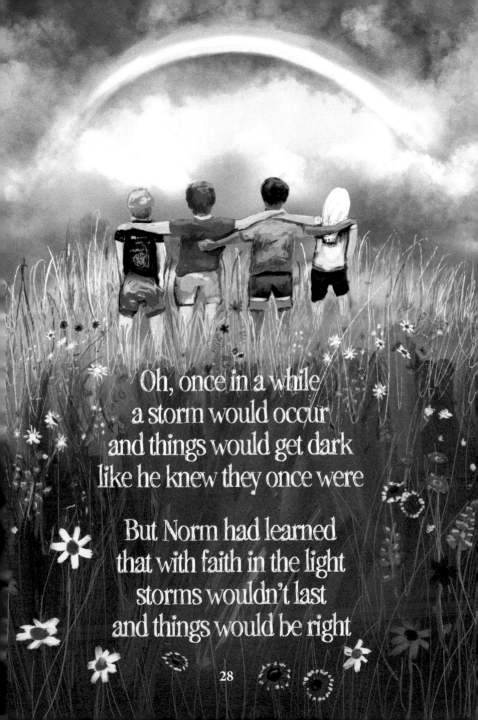

Oh, once in a while
a storm would occur
and things would get dark
like he knew they once were

But Norm had learned
that with faith in the light
storms wouldn't last
and things would be right

28

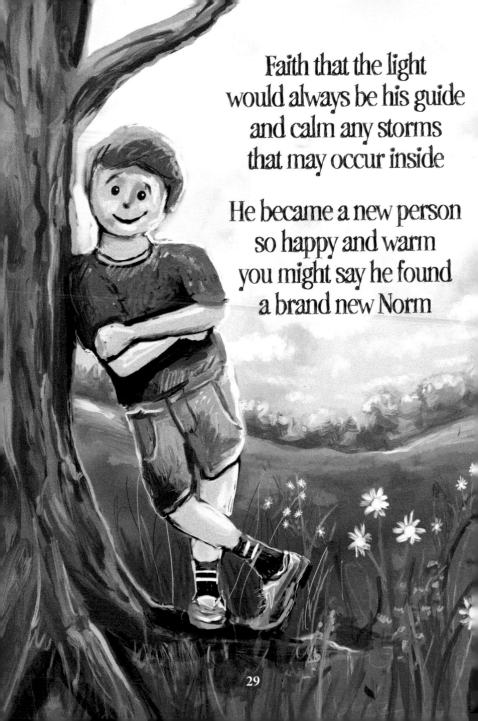

Faith that the light
would always be his guide
and calm any storms
that may occur inside

He became a new person
so happy and warm
you might say he found
a brand new Norm

The moral of this story
is within you there's a spark
with a yearning to grow
and overcome the dark

If you're willing to look
and focus on the good
you will find a better world
like you know the world could

Look not with your eyes
but with mind and heart
Let that be your normal
Let that be your start

What do you think?

"There once was a boy
whose name was Norm
and inside his head
was a terrible storm." (Page 1)

- What feelings do you have that are similar to Norm's?

- What situation in your life triggers that feeling?

- What about the situation can you control?

- If you could think about the situation differently, what would that thought be? How would your feelings change if you thought that way instead?

"He tried yelling and shouting
and screaming real loud
but it had no effect
on that nasty old cloud." (Page 15)

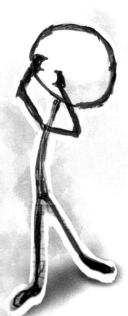

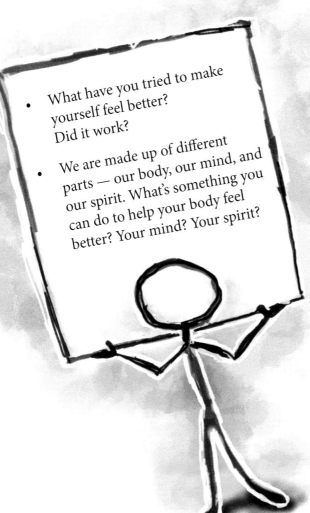

- What have you tried to make yourself feel better? Did it work?

- We are made up of different parts — our body, our mind, and our spirit. What's something you can do to help your body feel better? Your mind? Your spirit?

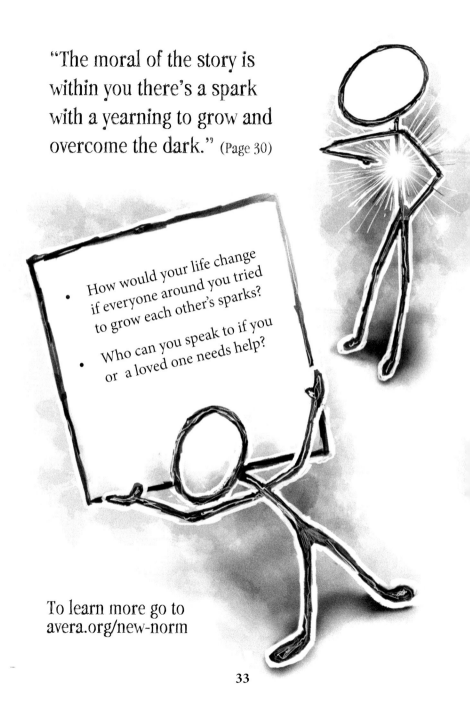

"The moral of the story is within you there's a spark with a yearning to grow and overcome the dark." (Page 30)

- How would your life change if everyone around you tried to grow each other's sparks?

- Who can you speak to if you or a loved one needs help?

To learn more go to avera.org/new-norm

The "spark of light" in the story, A New Norm, is intended to represent the positive essence that makes up the world around us, as well as the world within us. That light can be experienced in many forms, such as . . .

- Talking with an encouraging friend, family member, or trusted adult.
- Visiting with a counselor or therapist.
- Accepting professional medical help.
- Engaging in a healthy diet and exercise.
- Participating in creative activities.
- Helping others.
- Seeking a spiritual connection.

It is important to know that persistent negative thoughts can be very harmful both mentally and physically. Recognizing them and asking for help is the best way to start working toward a happier and healthier future.

What are some negative thoughts to be concerned about?

- Ongoing feelings of deep sadness.
- Always feeling anxious or upset.
- Sleeping too little or too much.
- Quick to anger or talking about seeking revenge.

If you, or someone you know, struggles with a cloud that may involve thoughts or behaviors like the ones above, please ask for help.

Call anytime day or night.
1-800-273-8255
Or Text HOME to 741741

Avera Behavioral Health: 1-800-691-4336

May you find your light and be well!

34

Tom & Tammy Roberts

A New Norm is author Tom Roberts'
seventh book created as a benefit for
Children's Home Society (CHS). Since
2002, Tom and Tammy have produced
*'Twas the Night Before Christ; Santa's
Prayer; The Little Lost Sock; Return To
The Farm; The Greatest Gift – The Wise
Ones Journey;* and his newest book,
On That One Christmas Eve. Over
the years Tom and Tammy have raised
awareness for CHS through a variety of storytelling presentations
and book signings, raising over $1.2 million to support the programs and services
that CHS offers to help kids and families across the state.

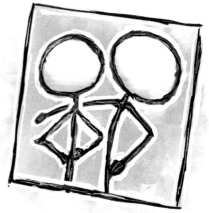

Jim Brummond

Jim Brummond is an artist, graphic designer,
illustrator, and photographer from Sioux Falls,
SD. He has been recognized locally, regionally,
and internationally with many awards
throughout his career.

This is the sixth book Jim has illustrated.
He is grateful to use his talents to help
people in need by designing and making art for several
area charities. "It truly is a great feeling to make the world a better place with
art, and I really enjoy knowing that by creating illustrations and designing this book,
I am helping kids and families!"

Avera ✠

Avera Health, based in Sioux Falls, SD, is an integrated health system across the Upper Midwest. As a health ministry rooted in the Gospel, Avera's mission is to make a positive impact in the lives and health of persons and communities by providing quality services guided by Christian values. Avera is a regional leader in behavioral health, with outpatient and inpatient programs for all ages and a full range of diagnoses including depression, anxiety, bipolar disorder, borderline personality disorder, dementia, schizophrenia, addiction, and more. Avera's world-class facilities provide specialized treatment for children, adolescents, adults, and seniors. For more information about Avera Health visit: Avera.org

CHILDREN'S HOME SOCIETY

Established in 1893, Children's Home Society (CHS) is the oldest human service nonprofit organization in South Dakota. CHS provides emergency shelter, residential treatment and special education, forensic interviews, foster care and adoption services, and prevention programs. In addition to serving victims of child abuse and domestic violence, CHS also partners with caring parents to help children with emotional or behavioral needs.

The CHS mission is to empower children, women, families, and communities to be resilient, safe, healthy, and strong.

For more Information about Children's Home Society visit: www.chssd.org

A Special Thanks to Our Sponsors

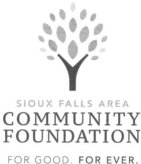

SIOUX FALLS AREA
COMMUNITY FOUNDATION
FOR GOOD. **FOR EVER.**

Avera Behavioral Health Center

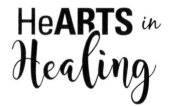

A special thanks to **Shantrel DeJong** who, as part of the Avera Team in the **Adolescent Group Therapy** department, was the "spark" that initiated the idea for this story. I would also like to thank the **Avera Clinical Team** who helped navigate this project. Thank you to our illustrator, **Jim Brummond**, for his patience, creativity, and artistic talent in bringing this story to life. And last, but not least, I'd like to thank **Tom and Laurie Chaplin** for their friendship and for providing an encouraging atmosphere in which to write this story.

–Tom Roberts